Trigeminal Ne

A Beginner's 3-Step Quick Start
TB Through Diet, With Sa

.....pes

Disclaimer

By reading this disclaimer, you are accepting the terms of the disclaimer in full. If you disagree with this disclaimer, please do not read the guide.

All of the content within this guide is provided for informational and educational purposes only, and should not be accepted as independent medical or other professional advice. The author is not a doctor, physician, nurse, mental health provider, or registered nutritionist/dietician. Therefore, using and reading this guide does not establish any form of a physician-patient relationship.

Always consult with a physician or another qualified health provider with any issues or questions you might have regarding any sort of medical condition. Do not ever disregard any qualified professional medical advice or delay seeking that advice because of anything you have read in this guide. The information in this guide is not intended to be any sort of medical advice and should not be used in lieu of any medical advice by a licensed and qualified medical professional.

The information in this guide has been compiled from a variety of known sources. However, the author cannot attest to or guarantee the accuracy of each source and thus should not be held liable for any errors or omissions.

Table of Contents

Introduction

Trigeminal neuralgia, also known as tic douloureux, is a condition that affects the trigeminal nerve, which is one of the cranial nerves. This nerve provides sensation to the face and controls many of the muscles in the face. Trigeminal neuralgia is caused by damage to the trigeminal nerve. This can be due to several things, including infection, a tumor, or trauma.

Symptoms of trigeminal neuralgia include sudden, sharp pain in the face that may be intermittent or constant. The pain may be on one side or both sides of the face, and it may vary in intensity. Other symptoms can include tingling or numbness in the face, drooping eyelids, and difficulty swallowing.

Trigeminal neuralgia is diagnosed based on a person's symptoms and medical history. A physical exam may also be done to look for signs of damage to the trigeminal nerve. Imaging tests such as MRI or CT scan may be done to help determine the cause of the trigeminal neuralgia.

There is no one-size-fits-all treatment for trigeminal neuralgia. Treatment options include medications, surgery, and home remedies. Medications can include painkillers and drugs that are used to treat seizures or nerve pain. Surgery may be needed if medications do not work or if there is damage to the trigeminal nerve.

Home remedies can include using ice packs or heat packs, avoiding triggers such as loud noises or strong smells, and adjusting your diet.

Managing trigeminal neuralgia can be difficult, but it is possible with patience and perseverance. It is important to work with your doctor to find a treatment plan that works for you.

In this beginner's guide, we'll discuss the following subtopics in further detail:

• What is the trigeminal nerve?

• What are the two types of trigeminal neuralgia?

• What causes trigeminal neuralgia?

• What are the symptoms of trigeminal neuralgia?

• Who is at risk to get trigeminal neuralgia?

• How is trigeminal neuralgia diagnosed?

• How is trigeminal neuralgia treated?

• Alternative treatments for trigeminal neuralgia.

• Managing trigeminal neuralgia through lifestyle changes.

• Managing trigeminal neuralgia through diet

• The 3-step guide to managing trigeminal neuralgia through diet and nutrition

Keep reading to know more about trigeminal neuralgia and how to manage this condition through diet.

What Is the Trigeminal Nerve?

The trigeminal nerve is the largest of the cranial nerves and is responsible for transmitting sensation from the face to the brain. It has three main branches: the ophthalmic nerve, the maxillary nerve, and the mandibular nerve.

Ophthalmic nerve: The ophthalmic nerve is the longest branching nerve of the trigeminal nerve. It innervates the skin of the forehead and scalp, as well as the conjunctiva and mucous membranes of the eye. The ophthalmic nerve gives rise to three main branches: the lacrimal nerve, the frontal nerve, and the nasociliary nerve.

• The lacrimal nerve innervates the lacrimal gland, which produces tears.

• The frontal nerve innervates the forehead.

• The nasociliary nerve innervates the nose and eye. It also gives rise to two smaller nerves: the infratrochlear nerve and the supratrochlear nerve. These nerves innervate the upper eyelid and eyebrow.

Maxillary nerve: The maxillary nerve is one of the three branches of the trigeminal nerve, and it innervates the skin of the upper lip and cheek, as well as the mucous membranes of the nose and palate. The maxillary nerve is responsible for sensation in these areas, as well as for the motor function of the muscles that control chewing. The maxillary nerve also gives rise to the zygomatic nerve, which innervates the muscles that raise the eyebrow.

Mandibular nerve: The mandibular nerve is the largest of the three nerves that arise from the trigeminal ganglion. It provides both motor and sensory innervation to the lower jaw, teeth, and skin of the lower lip and chin.

The motor fibers of the mandibular nerve innervate the muscles of mastication, which include the masseter, temporalis, medial pterygoid, and lateral pterygoid muscles. These muscles are responsible for chewing and grinding food.

The sensory fibers of the mandibular nerve provide sensation to the teeth, gingiva, mucous membranes, and skin of the lower lip and chin. In addition, the mandibular nerve also provides parasympathetic innervation to the salivary glands.

The trigeminal nerve also plays a role in mastication (chewing) by supplying motor fibers to the muscles of mastication. Lesions of the trigeminal nerve can cause facial pain, sensory loss, or motor paralysis.

What are the two types of trigeminal Neuralgia?

Trigeminal neuralgia is a chronic pain condition that affects the trigeminal nerve, which carries sensation from your face to your brain. There are two types of trigeminal neuralgia: classic (Type 1) and atypical (Type 2).

Classic trigeminal neuralgia: Classic TN is the more common type and is usually caused by compression of the trigeminal nerve by a blood vessel. Classic trigeminal neuralgia is characterized by sudden, severe, brief episodes of pain that feel like an electric shock. These episodes can happen without any trigger, or they can be triggered by activities like brushing your teeth or eating.

Atypical trigeminal neuralgia: Atypical TN is less common and is often caused by irritation of the trigeminal nerve by a tumor or multiple sclerosis. Atypical trigeminal neuralgia is characterized by sustained pain that is not as severe as classic trigeminal neuralgia. It may be triggered by light touch or contact with your hair, for example.

What Causes Trigeminal Neuralgia?

Trigeminal neuralgia (TN) is caused by compression or damage to the trigeminal nerve. This can be due to a variety of factors, including tumors, infections, injuries, and certain medical conditions.

• _Tumors:_ Tumors that grow in or around the trigeminal nerve can cause trigeminal neuralgia. These tumors can be benign (noncancerous) or malignant (cancerous).

• _Infections:_ Infections, such as shingles, that involve the trigeminal nerve can also lead to trigeminal neuralgia.

• _Injuries:_ Injuries to the head or face can damage the trigeminal nerve and lead to trigeminal neuralgia.

• _Medical conditions:_ Medical conditions that affect the nervous system, such as multiple sclerosis, can cause trigeminal neuralgia.

What are the symptoms of trigeminal neuralgia?

Pain in the parts of the face that are supplied by the trigeminal nerve is the most prominent sign that someone has trigeminal neuralgia. The pain is typically described as being intense, penetrating, or electrical. The pain can be so intense that it prevents a person from being able to eat, drink, talk, or even clean their teeth.

Trigeminal neuralgia sufferers typically experience a worsening of their discomfort when they are exposed to particular triggers, such as cleaning their teeth, eating, drinking, or talking. Even a light touch to your face might sometimes trigger discomfort. The discomfort may be intermittent or it may be consistent all the time.

Trigeminal neuralgia can cause pain that is so intense that it can in rare circumstances lead to sadness, anxiety, and even suicidal thoughts in some patients.

Who are at risk to get trigeminal neuralgia?

Several variables might put someone at risk for developing trigeminal neuralgia, including the following:

Age: Trigeminal neuralgia is a painful ailment that can affect anybody at any age; however, those over the age of 50 are most likely to suffer from it. Growing older brings with it an increased likelihood of experiencing trigeminal neuralgia.

Gender: The cause of the fact that trigeminal neuralgia affects women more frequently than it does men is not completely known. Alterations in hormone levels are one possible explanation for this phenomenon, which occurs when women reach menopause. There is also the possibility that it is connected to the higher rate of autoimmune illnesses that are seen in females.

Medical conditions: Diabetes, which can cause nerve damage over time, is considered to be one of the most prevalent factors that lead to trigeminal neuralgia. In addition to multiple sclerosis, cancer, and stroke, trigeminal neuralgia can also be caused by a variety of other medical disorders.

Trigeminal neuralgia is a debilitating ailment that can cause significant pain in the face and head. The exact source of this condition is unknown. It is essential to go to a medical professional to receive the most effective therapy for trigeminal neuralgia if you are afflicted with this condition. Numerous successful therapies are currently accessible, and with the assistance of a medical professional, you will be able to select the one that is most appropriate for you.

How Is Trigeminal Neuralgia Diagnosed?

A diagnosis of trigeminal neuralgia is often made after considering both the patient's symptoms and the results of a physical exam. In addition, your doctor may recommend certain tests, such as an MRI or CT scan, to rule out any potential other explanations for your discomfort.

Medical history and physical examination: The diagnosis of trigeminal neuralgia often begins with a thorough review of the patient's medical history as well as a physical examination. Your doctor will most likely ask you questions about your symptoms, including when they first appeared and what factors make them better or worse.

Imaging tests: Imaging tests could be required to rule out other illnesses that could be the source of symptoms that are quite similar in certain instances. These tests could involve computed tomography or magnetic resonance imaging (MRI), for example (CT). Electroneurography, often known as ENoG, may sometimes be utilized as well. The electrical activity of the trigeminal nerve is measured using this test, which can contribute to confirming the diagnosis.

Visit a medical professional as soon as possible if you have any reason to suspect that you could be suffering from trigeminal neuralgia. Only then will you be able to acquire an exact diagnosis and start the treatment process.

How Is Trigeminal Neuralgia Treated?

To alleviate the discomfort caused by trigeminal neuralgia, a variety of medications—both over-the-counter and prescription—may be used. These include anticonvulsants, antidepressants, and muscle relaxants. In rare instances, surgery can be required to release the pressure that is being placed on the trigeminal nerve.

Anticonvulsants: The electrical activity in the brain is brought under control by these drugs, which also stop seizures from occurring. Anticonvulsants including carbamazepine, phenytoin, and gabapentin are typically prescribed to patients. These drugs have the potential to be beneficial in relieving pain; however, they also have the potential to induce adverse effects such as drowsiness, nausea, and dizziness.

Antidepressants: Antidepressants are frequently used in the treatment of trigeminal neuralgia because of their ability to assist reduce pain by blocking the nerve fibers that transport pain signals to the brain. Trigeminal neuralgia is a painful condition that affects the face and jaw. In addition, antidepressants can assist to enhance both a person's mood and the quality of their sleep, both of which can contribute to a reduction in the amount of pain experienced.

There are several various formulations of antidepressants available, and the one that works best for an individual will vary from case to case. As a result, it is essential to collaborate with a healthcare expert to select the most appropriate course of therapy.

Muscle relaxants: One type of medication that may be helpful in the treatment of this illness is known as muscle relaxants. These medications alleviate pain by calming muscular spasms, which is one of their primary mechanisms of action. Relaxants for the muscles are normally consumed by the mouth, but they can also be injected directly into the afflicted region. The usage of muscle relaxants can cause sleepiness, dizziness, and nausea as unwanted side effects.

Botox injection: Injections of Botox may potentially be used to give relief from the discomfort caused by trigeminal neuralgia. The facial muscles are paralyzed as a result of the injections, which eliminates any possibility of the muscles causing discomfort. Injections of Botox can help reduce the activity of the trigeminal nerve, which in turn helps avoid recurrent episodes of the painful condition known as trigeminal neuralgia. As a consequence of this, receiving injections of Botox for the treatment of this ailment that causes chronic pain is both risk-free and productive.

Surgery: Even though there are many other methods of therapy available, surgery is frequently the most successful choice. There are two primary categories of surgery that are used to treat trigeminal neuralgia, and they are microvascular decompression and radiofrequency ablation.

• *Microvascular decompression:* The most common type of surgical therapy for trigeminal neuralgia is referred to as microvascular decompression. The trigeminal nerve will be given some breathing room during this operation so that it can heal properly. A teeny-tiny pad or sponge is attached to the nerve to do this. This cushion shields the nerve from any potential pressure that may be coming from the blood vessels. In certain instances, the surgeon could also be required to cut away a minute portion of bone. Microvascular decompression surgery is a more intrusive procedure; nevertheless, it has a greater potential to provide long-term relief. This operation has a success rate that varies from sixty to eighty percent of the time.

• *Radiofrequency ablation:* Ablation using radiofrequency is less intrusive than other methods, but it may require many sessions over time to keep working well. Radio waves are used in this method to generate heat in the trigeminal nerve. Because of this, the nerve gets damaged, and as a result, it is unable to transmit pain signals to the brain. Radiofrequency ablation is a less intrusive treatment option than microvascular decompression; nevertheless, it also has a lower success rate. A success rate of between 30 and 50 percent might be expected with radiofrequency ablation.

Even though surgery has the potential to be a successful therapy for trigeminal neuralgia, there are certain dangers associated with the procedure. Infection, hemorrhage, and numbness in the face are the most prevalent types of problems that might arise. Anesthesia-related problems are a possibility, as they are with any type of surgical procedure. However, many people can find relief from the pain caused by trigeminal neuralgia if they receive the appropriate care and therapy.

However, regardless of the method that is chosen for therapy, the primary objective is to lessen the amount of discomfort that the patient is in. Even though there is no known cure for trigeminal neuralgia, the majority of people can find considerable relief from their pain with the right therapy.

Alternative treatments for trigeminal neuralgia

Trigeminal neuralgia is a painful condition that may be managed with medicine and surgery, but various alternative treatments can be helpful. The following are some of these:

Acupuncture: A procedure that is used in traditional Chinese medicine called acupuncture involves placing very thin needles into precise points on the skin at various locations. It is believed that doing this will activate the nerve system, which in turn may assist ease pain.

Massage: The muscles and soft tissues that are located close to the trigeminal nerve can be worked on during massage treatment to provide pain relief. It may also help reduce stress and tension, both of which may contribute to the onset of pain episodes or trigger existing ones worse.

Yoga: Because it helps to increase blood circulation and reduce inflammation, yoga may be beneficial for those suffering from trigeminal neuralgia. It has also been demonstrated to be effective in helping to alleviate tension and anxiety, both of which can make the pain seem much worse.

Diet and nutrition: Even though medicine is the most prevalent method of treatment for TN, there are other forms of treatment, such as food and nutrition, that may be helpful to certain people who have the condition. In addition to changes in diet, the inclusion of some vitamins could also assist to alleviate discomfort.

Biofeedback: You may get relief from the discomfort caused by trigeminal neuralgia by utilizing biofeedback as an alternate form of therapy. The process of learning to manage your body's physiological reaction to discomfort can be accomplished through biofeedback. You can learn to lessen muscular tension and other physical symptoms linked with trigeminal neuralgia by using biofeedback. These symptoms include facial pain and headaches.

In certain circumstances, biofeedback has the potential to potentially avert the development of painful sensations. Talk to your primary care physician about getting a referral to a qualified biofeedback practitioner if you are interested in investigating the possibility of using biofeedback as a therapy for trigeminal neuralgia.

Chiropractic care: The manipulation of the spine and other portions of the body that is involved in chiropractic therapy is intended to reduce pain and promote healing.

Each of these treatments has the potential to offer patients suffering from trigeminal neuralgia some degree of comfort, and they may also assist to enhance the patient's overall quality of life.

Managing Trigeminal Neuralgia Through Lifestyle Changes

Changes to one's lifestyle, when used as part of a pain management strategy for trigeminal neuralgia, can be highly successful.

Proper washing of face: One of the most helpful things you can do to treat trigeminal neuralgia is to wash your face with warm water. Some people believe that using warm water is preferable since, unlike hot water, it does not cause their skin to get irritated.

In addition, the use of cold water can cause the blood vessels in the face to contract, which can make the discomfort seem much worse. Make sure to use a mild cleanser that won't irritate your skin when you wash your face with warm water. This will prevent your skin from losing its natural oils. Scrubs and exfoliants that are too abrasive should also be avoided since they might aggravate existing skin irritation.

Eating the right foods: Eating foods that are soft and avoiding liquids that are either hot or cold can help prevent the onset of painful episodes. In addition to this, it is essential to have a nutritious diet overall. This entails consuming a diet that is abundant in fruits, vegetables, whole grains, and lean sources of protein. Eating a diet low in saturated fat, high in fruits and vegetables, and moderate in protein can assist to minimize pain and inflammation, and will also help to increase your general health.

Avoid trigger foods: Although trigeminal neuralgia does not have a known cure, there are treatments available that can help control the pain and lessen both the frequency and severity of attacks. Avoiding the foods that trigger your allergies is one strategy. Spicy foods, coffee, salty, acidic, and hot beverages are common examples of things that might set off an allergic reaction.

If you suffer from trigeminal neuralgia, it is important to pay attention to what you eat and drink, and you should make an effort to steer clear of any items that seem to exacerbate your symptoms. You might also find it helpful to consult with a qualified dietitian about other dietary adjustments that could be able to assist you in better managing your pain.

Good oral care: After eating, it might be helpful to give your mouth a thorough rinsing with water at room temperature and brush your teeth gently with a toothbrush that has soft bristles. This can be an effective aspect of a management strategy for trigeminal neuralgia.

Quit smoking: Stopping smoking is one of the most beneficial things you can do for your health if you are a smoker. Tobacco smoking is linked to an increase in both chronic pain and inflammation, in addition to a host of other major health issues. Talk to your primary care physician about getting help to kick the habit of smoking if you suffer from trigeminal neuralgia.

Manage stress: The discomfort caused by trigeminal neuralgia might be made worse by stress. Finding effective ways to handle stress will help you feel better overall and may even make it possible for you to avoid future pain episodes. There are many various approaches to managing stress, including yoga, meditation, and relaxation therapies like yoga and meditation. Find the approach that serves you most effectively, and then stay with it.

Exercise: The management of trigeminal neuralgia also includes the use of exercise as an important component. Exercising can help you feel less stressed, enhance your general health, and boost your ability to tolerate discomfort for longer periods. It is essential to locate a physical activity routine that is suitable for you and to maintain it consistently. If you have never exercised before, it is recommended that you discuss starting carefully with your primary care provider.

Get enough sleep: To effectively manage trigeminal neuralgia, enough sleep is necessary. Insomnia can exacerbate discomfort and make it more difficult to deal with the disease you're already dealing with. Always aim to obtain at least eight hours of sleep each night, and make it a priority to maintain as much of a consistent sleeping pattern as you possibly can.

Identify trigger factors: If you are aware that the wind is one of the factors that contribute to your discomfort, consider wrapping a scarf lightly over your face while it is windy and wearing it over your face. Additionally, you should make an effort to steer clear of any elements known to bring on episodes of pain in the past.

You might be able to enhance your quality of life and experience less pain if you adopt any of these lifestyle adjustments and give them some thought.

Managing Trigeminal Neuralgia Through Diet

As was just discussed, nutrition is an essential factor to consider while trying to manage trigeminal neuralgia. The following are some particular dietary suggestions that may be of assistance:

The Low Saturated Fat Diet

Inflammation, which may cause pain and other health problems, can spread throughout the body when a person consumes a diet that is high in saturated fats. It may be possible to alleviate pain and inflammation by lowering the quantity of saturated fat consumed in one's diet. In addition to other sources of saturated fat, processed meats and full-fat dairy products are examples of foods that have a high concentration of unhealthy fat known as saturated fat.

It may be possible to alleviate pain and inflammation by avoiding or restricting the consumption of certain foods. Instead, you should make it a priority to consume a greater quantity of lean meats, chicken, fish, tofu, legumes, nuts, seeds, and healthy oils. These meals have a reduced percentage of saturated fat and have been shown to help decrease pain and inflammation in the body.

You can assist to alleviate the pain and inflammation produced by trigeminal neuralgia by incorporating these dietary adjustments into your routine.

The Mediterranean Diet

The Mediterranean diet is a way of eating that emphasizes consuming a variety of fresh fruits and vegetables, as well as whole grains, seafood, and olive oil. It has been demonstrated that this particular diet can lessen both pain and inflammation. The foods that have been eaten for generations in Mediterranean nations like Greece, Italy, and Spain form the basis of the diet known as the Mediterranean diet.

High consumption of fruits, vegetables, whole grains, seafood, and olive oil are the primary tenets of this eating plan. These foods include a high concentration of antioxidants and other substances that have anti-inflammatory properties, which may contribute to a reduction in pain and inflammation. In addition, following a diet similar to that of the Mediterranean has been linked to a lower chance of developing chronic illnesses such as coronary heart disease, cancer, and Alzheimer's disease.

Therefore, adopting a diet similar to that of the Mediterranean may provide several positive effects on one's health. The Mediterranean diet is a wonderful choice to explore if you are thinking about making adjustments to your diet to alleviate the pain associated with trigeminal neuralgia.

The 3-Step Guide to Managing Trigeminal Neuralgia Through Diet and Nutrition

No one diet is guaranteed to alleviate the symptoms of trigeminal neuralgia in every single patient, but following certain general dietary guidelines might help reduce pain and inflammation.

Step 1. Eliminate trigger foods: Eliminating the foods that act as triggers is the first step in treating trigeminal neuralgia through dietary modifications, just as it is the first step in managing other lifestyle adjustments. Spicy foods, coffee, salty, acidic, and hot beverages are common examples of things that might set off an allergic reaction. If you suffer from trigeminal neuralgia, it is important to pay attention to what you eat and drink, and you should make an effort to steer clear of any items that seem to exacerbate your symptoms.

• *Spicy foods*: Consuming particularly spicy foods might aggravate nerve discomfort and perhaps cause the nerve to become inflamed. If you suffer from trigeminal neuralgia, it is in your best interest to steer clear of foods that are particularly hot or to consume them with extreme caution.

• _Coffee:_ The chemicals included in coffee have the potential to irritate the trigeminal nerve. For example, caffeine is a known migraine trigger, and a significant number of patients who suffer from trigeminal neuralgia also get migraines. In addition, the temperature of the coffee, which is often served hot, is another factor that might bring on an episode of trigeminal neuralgia. As a consequence of this, it is essential for persons who have this illness to be aware of the potential triggers and to steer clear of them to the greatest extent that they can.

• _Salty foods:_ Because it causes inflammation, salt may be a source of discomfort. Even the smallest of motions can produce excruciating pain if the trigeminal nerve is irritated. If you have trigeminal neuralgia, you must stay away from foods that are high in salt for this reason. Although limiting salt won't make the illness go away, doing so may make uncomfortable flare-ups less likely to occur.

• _Acidic foods:_ As another potential source of discomfort, acidic foods can be irritating to the trigeminal nerve. If you suffer from trigeminal neuralgia, you should thus make it a point to steer clear of foods that are high in acidity. Citrus fruits, tomatoes, vinegar, and coffee are some of the most popular foods that fall into the category of acidic foods. These foods are known to be pain triggers. If you discover that consuming acidic foods is making your discomfort worse, consider cutting them out of your diet entirely or eating them in much smaller quantities.

• _Hot beverages:_ Drinks that are too hot might cause pain by irritating the trigeminal nerve. If you suffer from trigeminal neuralgia, you should steer clear of drinking hot liquids or consuming them with extreme caution.

Step 2. Include anti-inflammatory foods: Incorporating foods that are known to lower inflammation and pain is yet another dietary strategy that may be of assistance to a person in need of such relief. Omega-3 fatty acids, herbs, spices like ginger and turmeric, and dark leafy greens are some examples of these.

• _Omega-3 fatty acids:_ Omega-3 fatty acids are a kind of fat that has been shown to reduce inflammation in the body. Walnuts, flaxseeds, and chia seeds are all good sources of omega-3 fatty acids, as are oily seafood like salmon, mackerel, and sardines. If you want to experience less pain and inflammation, adding these items to your diet might help.

• _Herbs and spices:_ Ginger and turmeric are only two examples of herbs and spices that have anti-inflammatory qualities. It's possible that including them in your diet can help you feel less pain and inflammation.

• _Dark leafy greens:_ In addition to being rich in vitamins and minerals, dark leafy greens like spinach and kale also contain anthocyanins, which are compounds that reduce inflammation. It's possible that including them in your diet can help you feel less pain and experience less inflammation.

Step 3. Consider supplements: Alterations to one's diet can be helpful for persons who suffer from trigeminal neuralgia; nevertheless, some patients also find relief from taking supplements. Magnesium, vitamins B6 and B12, and omega-3 fatty acids are all examples of dietary supplements that might be beneficial.

• _Magnesium:_ Magnesium is a mineral that is useful in the treatment of painful conditions. You can get it in the form of dietary supplements or foods like chocolates with a high cocoa content, legumes, nuts, and seeds.

• _Vitamins B6 and B12:_ These vitamins are important components of the neurological system and have been shown to effectively alleviate pain. They are available as dietary supplements as well as in foods including beef, chicken, fish, eggs, and dairy products.

• _Omega-3 fatty acids:_ As was discussed earlier, omega-3 fatty acids are a form of fat that possesses qualities that make it effective against inflammation. They are available as dietary supplements as well as in foods like walnuts, oily salmon, flaxseeds, and chia seeds, among others.

Before making any modifications to your diet to alleviate the symptoms of trigeminal neuralgia, you must discuss your options with a certified dietitian or another qualified healthcare professional. They can assist you in formulating a strategy that caters to your unique requirements and offer advice on how to implement adjustments that are practical for your lifestyle.

Making adjustments to one's lifestyle, such as altering one's food, can be an efficient method of pain management and reduction when dealing with trigeminal neuralgia. Have a conversation with a qualified dietitian or another healthcare expert to formulate a strategy that is tailored specifically to your needs.

Sample Recipes

<u>Arugula and Mushroom Salad</u>

Ingredients:

• 5 oz. arugula washed

• 1 lb. fresh mushrooms

• 1/4 tsp. shoyu

• 1/2 red onion

• 1 tbsp. olive oil

• 1 tbsp. mirin

For tofu cheese:

• 1/8 cup umeboshi vinegar

• 1/2 firm tofu

Instructions:

1. In a bowl, add the rinsed tofu. Crumble and pour in vinegar.

2. In a separate bowl add shoyu, red onions, salt, olive oil, and mirin. 3. Mix to combine.

4. Add in the arugula and toss to combine with the dressing.

5. Serve and enjoy.

Mediterranean Vegetables

Ingredients:

• 16 oz. mixed frozen broccoli, carrots, and cauliflower

• 1 tbsp. drained capers

• 1 can diced tomatoes, basil, garlic, and oregano

Instructions:

1. Combine tomatoes, mixed vegetables, and drained capers in a microwave-safe bowl.

2. Cover with plastic wrap.

3. Bake for 6 to 8 minutes on high heat.

4. Stir halfway.

5. Serve and enjoy.

Green Coleslaw

Ingredients:

- 1/2 cup white distilled vinegar

- 1/4 cup granulated white sugar

- 1 tsp. kosher salt

- 1/4 tsp. black pepper

- 1/2 head green cabbage shredded

Instructions:

1. Stir together vinegar, sugar, salt, and pepper until well combined and sugar is dissolved.

2. Place cabbage in a large bowl and pour vinegar mixture over it.

3. Stir to combine.

4. Let coleslaw sit for at least 30 minutes at room temperature, to let the flavors meld.

5. Serve with pulled pork, BBQ chicken, fish tacos, or as a side for a grilled feast.

Grilled Macrobiotic Bowl with Stir Fry Broccoli, Onions, and Carrots

Ingredients:

- 2 tbsp. garlic, minced

- 2 tbsp. olive oil

- 1/2 cup adzuki beans cooked

- 1/2 cup sauerkraut

- 1 cup quinoa

- 1/2 cup cubed butternut squash

- 1 tbsp. dulse flakes

- 1 1/2 cup baby kale

- 1 tbsp. toasted pumpkin seeds

- salt

- pepper

Garlic Cashew Creme:

- 3 cloves garlic

- 1/2 cup raw cashews

- 1 lemon, juice only

- 1/2 tsp. sea salt

Instructions:

1. Add the butternut to a large glass bowl to pre-cook for 2 minutes.

2. On the grill, spread some olive oil. Add rice, butternut, sauerkraut, greens, and beans.

3. For 5 to 7 minutes, grill on medium-high, turning the ingredients frequently until cooked.

4. Sprinkle a dash of salt and pepper to taste.

5. To make the garlic cashew creme, blend all ingredients in a high-speed blender; set aside.

6. Assemble the bowl by sprinkling dulse flakes and toasted pumpkin seeds and top with garlic cashew creme.

Asian Zucchini Salad

Ingredients:

• 1 medium zucchini, sliced thinly into spirals

• 1/3 cup rice vinegar

• 3/4 cup avocado oil

• 1 cup sunflower seeds, shells removed

• 1 lb. cabbage, shredded

• 1 tsp. stevia drops

• 1 cup almonds, sliced

Instructions:

1. Cut the zucchini spirals into smaller parts. Set aside.

2. Put almonds, sunflower seeds, and cabbage in a large bowl. Combine the ingredients well.

4. Add zucchini to the mixture.

5. In a small bowl, mix vinegar, stevia, and oil using a whisk or fork.

6. Pour the vinegar mixture all over the zucchini mixture. Toss well. Make sure everything is covered with the dressing.

7. Refrigerate for 2 hours before serving.

Baked Salmon

Ingredients:

• 2 salmon fillets

• 6 cups of fresh spinach

• 2 tsp. coconut oil

• 1/4 tsp. garlic powder

• 1/4 tsp. turmeric

• 3 large cloves of garlic

• lemon juice

• salt

• pepper

Instructions:

1. Preheat the oven to 400°F.

2. Line a baking dish with parchment paper.

3. Marinate salmon fillets in lemon juice, coconut oil, garlic powder, turmeric, salt, and pepper.

4. Let it sit for a few minutes. This may also be done the night before to help the juices and flavor get into the salmon.

5. Once the oven is ready, bake the salmon for 15 minutes.

6. Cook some of the garlic in a pan with coconut oil.

7. Add spinach and cook until ready. Season with salt and pepper to taste.

8. Take salmon out of the oven and put spinach beside it.

9. Serve and enjoy.

Lemon-Baked Salmon

Ingredients:

- 2 pcs. lemons, thinly sliced
- 3 lbs. salmon filet
- kosher salt
- black pepper, freshly ground
- 6 tbsp. butter, melted, 6 tbsp.
- 2 tbsp. honey
- 3 cloves garlic, minced
- 1 tsp. thyme leaves, chopped
- 1 tsp. dried oregano
- fresh parsley, chopped, for garnish

Instructions:

1. Preheat the oven to 350°F.

2. Line a rimmed baking sheet with foil. Grease with cooking oil spray.

3. Lay lemon slices on the center of the foil.

4. Season salmon filets on both sides with kosher salt and freshly ground black pepper.

5. Place the filet on top of the lemon slices.

6. Whisk together oregano, thyme, garlic, honey, and butter in a small bowl.

7. Pour the mixture over the salmon filet.

8. Fold the foil up and around the salmon to form a packet.

9. Bake for 25 minutes or until the salmon is cooked through.

10. Switch to broil and continue cooking for 2 more minutes.

11. Garnish with chopped fresh parsley and serve hot.

Asparagus and Greens Salad with Tahini and Poppy Seed Dressing

Ingredients:

• 10 to 12 asparagus stalks, washed well and sliced into ribbons

• 5 radishes, washed well and sliced thinly

• 2 to 3 rainbow carrots, peeled and sliced thinly

• 1 handful of wild spinach

• 1 small handful of microgreens, washed well

• 1 small handful of sunflower greens, washed well

• optional: a few pieces of chive blossoms

For the dressing:

• 2 tbsp. tahini

• 1 tbsp. poppy seeds

• 1 tbsp. extra-virgin olive oil

• salt

• pepper

Instructions:

1. For the dressing, whisk ingredients together in a small bowl.

2. In a separate bowl, toss salad ingredients into the mixture.

3. Drizzle dressing on salad upon serving.

Salmon with Avocados and Brussels Sprouts

Ingredients:

• 2 lbs. of salmon filet, divided into 4 pieces

• 1 tsp. ground cumin

• 1 tsp. onion powder

• 1 tsp. paprika powder

• 1/2 tsp. garlic powder

• 1 tsp. chili powder

• Himalayan sea salt

• black pepper, freshly ground

Avocado sauce:

• 2 chopped avocados

• 1 lime, squeezed for the juice

• 1 tbsp. extra-virgin olive oil

• 1 tbsp. fresh minced cilantro

• 1 diced small red onion

• 1 minced garlic clove

• Himalayan sea salt to taste

• black pepper, freshly ground

Brussels sprouts:

• 3 lbs. of Brussels sprouts

- 1/2 cup raw honey

- 1/2 cup balsamic vinegar

- 1/2 cup melted coconut oil

- 1 cup dried cranberries

- Himalayan sea salt

- black pepper, freshly ground

Instructions:

To make the salmon and avocado sauce:

1. Combine cumin, onion, chili powder, garlic, and paprika seasoned with salt and pepper. Mix well before dry rubbing on the salmon.

2. Place the salmon in the fridge for 30 minutes.

3. Preheat the grill.

4. In a bowl, mash avocado until the texture becomes smooth. Pour in all the remaining ingredients and mix thoroughly.

5. Grill salmon for 5 minutes on each side or until cooked.

6. Drizzle avocado on cooked salmon.

To make the Brussel Sprout:

1. Preheat the oven to 375°F.

2. Mix Brussels sprouts with coconut oil. Season with salt and pepper.

3. Place vegetables on a baking sheet and roast for about 30 minutes.

4. In a separate pan, combine vinegar and honey.

5. Simmer in slow heat until it boils and thickens.

6. Drizzle them on top of the Brussels sprouts.

7. Serve with the salmon.

Support for Trigeminal Neuralgia Patients

Many others share your experience of living with trigeminal neuralgia. There is a wide variety of support groups and organizations available, each with the ability to supply beneficial information and resources. The Trigeminal Neuralgia Association is one example of this type of organization (TNA). The TNA hosts regular meetings of support groups, distributes educational resources, and hosts an annual conference.

If you know someone who suffers from trigeminal neuralgia, it is in everyone's best interest to assist them in any manner that you can. This involves having an awareness of the disease, providing emotional support, and offering assistance with day-to-day activities as required. Pain from trigeminal neuralgia can frequently cause patients to have mental health issues such as anxiety and depression. It is imperative that you support your friend or loved one by being there for them through these challenging moments.

Trigeminal neuralgia can make daily life challenging, but there are techniques to cope with the disease and resources available to provide help. Have a discussion about your choices with a medical professional, and look into support groups and other organizations that might be able to assist you.

References

Diet therapy for trigeminal neuralgia – SAPNA Pain Management Blog. (2019, February 4). Spine and Pain Clinics of North America. https://www.sapnamed.com/blog/diet-therapy-for-trigeminal-neuralgia/.

ePainAssist, T. (2019, July 6). What foods should you avoid & eat if you have trigeminal neuralgia? Epainassist. https://www.epainassist.com/diet-and-nutrition/what-foods-should-you-avoid-and-eat-if-you-have-trigeminal-neuralgia.

How watching your diet works wonders in managing trigeminal neuralgia. (n.d.). Retrieved October 27, 2022, from https://www.manilachiropractor.com/blog/539164-how-watching-your-diet-works-wonders-in-managing-trigeminal-neuralgia.

Microvascular decompression. (n.d.). Ucsfhealth.Org. Retrieved October 27, 2022, from https://www.ucsfhealth.org/treatments/microvascular%20decompression.

Trigeminal neuralgia: Symptoms, causes, treatment & surgery. (n.d.). Cleveland Clinic. Retrieved October 27, 2022, from

https://my.clevelandclinic.org/health/diseases/15671
-trigeminal-neuralgia-tn.

Trigeminal neuralgia. (2021, September 29).
https://www.hopkinsmedicine.org/health/conditions
-and-diseases/trigeminal-neuralgia.

Trigeminal neuralgia. (n.d.). Body Fabulous Natural
Health Clinic. Retrieved October 27, 2022, from
https://www.mybodyfabulous.co.uk/health/2016/11/
2/trigeminal-neuralgia.

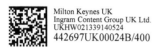

9 781088 111888